The Breastfeeding Parent

Nurturing, Loving, and Bonding

Table of Contents

Chapter 1. Introduction

Introducing a heartfelt exploration of an amazingly intimate journey in our Special Report: "The Breastfeeding Parent: Nurturing, Loving, and Bonding." This report beautifully captures the exceptional bond formed in the simple, yet profoundly magical act of breastfeeding. Delving into the realms of nurturing, it highlights the role played by this natural process in building an unshakable foundation of love and attachment between parent and child. Enlivened with personal narratives, expert insights, and the latest research findings, it illuminates the physical and emotional benefits that breastfeeding can bring. Intrigued? Open up to a world of boundless love and deep-rooted connection like never before with our Special Report. Be ready to discover, learn, and be inspired!

Chapter 2. The Powerful Bond: Understanding the Science Behind Breastfeeding and Attachment

Breastfeeding forms the cradle of emotional affection and connection, and it's time to marvel at the Science behind this unparalleled bond sculpted in nature's workshop.

2.1. The Biological Chemistry

Breastfeeding is not just simply feeding; nature has intricately engineered it to be a cauldron of a variety of chemicals that work their magic to create an indelible bond. Let's explore the biochemistry, a riveting tale of 'nature's love potion.'

The key components here are a set of chemicals known as hormones. Hormones such as prolactin and oxytocin are involved in the process of breastfeeding and also profoundly impact the emotional state of the nursing parent.

Prolactin, responsible for milk production, not only satiates hunger, but it also provides an enormous amount of sensory pleasure. Born out of suckling, prolactin washes over the breastfeeding parent and typically brings feelings of peace and contentment along, thereby letting them enjoy the act of nursing and bond with their baby.

Oxytocin, popularly known as the 'love hormone,' plays a crucial role during labor and continues its magic during the breastfeeding period. It encourages nurturing and protective behavior and oversees attachment, making it a significant catalyst in the bonding process.

2.2. The Role of Skin-to-Skin Contact

Often times during breastfeeding, babies are held close, belly-to-belly, skin-to-skin. This proximity allows them to smell the parent, hear their heartbeat and warmth, all of which contributes to creating a sense of security.

Skin-to-skin contact often results in the baby and the parent having coordinated heart rates and body temperatures. Research indicates that such synchrony could foster emotional tuning, laying the groundwork for developing empathy. The more skin-to-skin contact the baby has, the stronger this influence becomes.

This nurturing connection provides an environment where a baby feels safe, secure, and understood, and is crucial in the development of the brain's social and emotional networks.

2.3. Breastmilk: A Natural Comforter

Breastmilk is nature's remarkable produce, packed with nutrients and antibodies, but it's also something more. During nursing, babies receive 'comfort' through breastmilk that helps soothe and calm them.

The composition of breastmilk changes not only from day to day but throughout each feeding, responding to the baby's needs. For example, if a baby is unwell, the composition of the breastmilk changes to increase disease-fighting components. This dynamic system provides not only the physical comfort of satiety but also the emotional comfort of receiving precisely what the body needs at any given moment.

This miraculous adaptation of breastmilk is, in itself, a form of communication. This 'liquid love' sends a clear, comforting message to the baby: "You're taken care of."

2.4. Significance in a Larger Framework

Breastfeeding weaves a durable tapestry of secure attachment, a crucial element in a child's long-term emotional and social development. The bond fostered during breastfeeding creates a secure base for the child to explore the world and a lasting sense of trust in their caregivers.

Being consistently responsive to a baby's cues builds feelings of safety and security in the infant, promotes optimal brain development, and lays the foundation for a healthy sense of self-worth and empathy toward others.

2.5. The Power of Presence

Breastfeeding demands the full presence of the caregiver, from observing the baby's early hunger cues to responding appropriately to their needs. Regularly meeting a baby's needs creates a rhythm and predictability, giving them a sense of safety and trust in the world.

Nurturing presence is a gift that extends beyond the act of breastfeeding itself. It is an offering of emotional sustenance that enriches the relationship between parent and child, fostering emotional resilience. The breastfeeding journey, however, is not just about the physical sustenance but is deeply rooted in emotional connection that flourishes over time.

In conclusion, understanding the science behind breastfeeding and attachment makes it evident that breastfeeding is much more than a simple act of feeding. It is an intricate choreography of hormonal interactions, skin-to-skin contact, and psychological attunement that fortifies a foundation of secure attachment, thereby nurturing an everlasting bond of love and nurturing care between the parent and baby. It truly illustrates the phrase "the personal is biological," demonstrating how deeply our bodies and minds are interconnected in this intimate dance of nurturing.

Chapter 3. Breastfeeding Basics: A Comprehensive Guide for New Parents

Breastfeeding, a miracle of nature that has sustained life for countless generations, is an intimate process with a myriad of benefits for both parent and child. Establishing a successful breastfeeding relationship can often be a matter of knowledge and practice. This comprehensive guide is compiled to assist new parents in mastering the basics of this important journey.

3.1. The Physiology of Breastfeeding

Breastfeeding operates on a simple principle of supply and demand. Your body is designed to produce milk in response to your baby's feeding signal, which is primarily sucking. Hormones such as prolactin and oxytocin play a major role in milk production and release. Your breasts will produce colostrum, the first milk, right after giving birth, which is rich in antibodies, nutrients and minerals essential for your baby. As time progresses, your milk will change to be fuller and richer to cater to your baby's growing needs.

3.2. Preparing for Breastfeeding

Breastfeeding might seem challenging at first, but preparation can make it easier. For mothers, focusing on a nutritive diet, minimal stress levels, and adequate hydration can improve milk production. Understanding breastfeeding positions is also a great preparatory step. You can practise these positions with a doll or a pillow, switching between cradle-hold, cross-cradle hold, football hold, and side-lying position to find what might be most comfortable for you.

3.3. Latching: The Key to Successful Breastfeeding

Latching refers to how your baby attaches itself to your breast during feedings. A good latch ensures that your baby can effectively get milk from your breast, keeping nipple pain to a minimum. Signs of a good latch include more areola visible above your baby's upper lip than the lower lip, the baby's lips flanged outwards, rhythmic and deep sucks, and feeling of comfort while feeding.

3.4. Common Breastfeeding Positions

There are various positions to breastfeed, and it can require some time to find what works best for you and your baby. Some of the most common positions include:

- **Cradle Hold**: This traditional position involves cradling your baby across your chest, with the baby's head resting on your forearm.

- **Cross-Cradle Hold**: Similar to the cradle hold, this position allows you to have more control of your baby's head, which can be useful for new parents or parents with small infants.

- **Football Hold**: As the name suggests, you hold your baby like a football, tucked under your arm. This position can be beneficial for mothers who've had a C-section or with large breasts.

- **Side-Lying Position**: In this position, both you and the baby lie down facing each other. This can be a comfortable position for nighttime feedings.

Always remember to switch sides between feedings or in the middle of feedings to ensure both breasts are emptied, reducing the risk of engorgement, blocked ducts, or mastitis.

3.5. Navigating Common Breastfeeding Challenges

Many new parents worry about breastfeeding problems but knowing what might come your way makes it less daunting. Some common challenges include sore nipples, engorged breasts, low milk supply and mastitis. If you face these issues, remember that reaching out to a lactation consultant can help. Simple measures like using a suitable nipple cream, using warm compresses for engorgement, nursing frequently for boosting milk supply, and seeking prompt medical attention for mastitis can go a long way.

3.6. The Benefits of Breastfeeding

The benefits of breastfeeding extend far beyond nutrition. Breast milk contains several antibodies helping in building your baby's immune system. It also changes as your baby grows to meet the changing nutritional needs. From the mother's perspective, breastfeeding can help in losing pregnancy weight more quickly, can help in reducing the risk of breast and ovarian cancer, and even build a stronger bond with her baby.

Breastfeeding is a journey of unmatched intimacy and love. It may have its challenges, but it brings unparalleled rewards. Remember, there's no 'perfect' way to breastfeed and what matters the most is ensuring both you and your baby are comfortable. So embark on this journey armed with knowledge, patience, and heaps of love.

Chapter 4. From Birth to Weaning: Navigating Stages of Breastfeeding

It's the moment new parents both anticipate and cherish – the first time their newborn latches on. It can also be a time of apprehension. But, as many breastfeeding parents will tell you, with patience, support, and commitment, these early moments can bloom into a beautiful bonding experience that ultimately nurtures a lasting mother-child bond.

4.1. The First Hours

Immediately after birth, a time when both parent and infant are recovering from the quite literally life-changing experience of birth, it's encouraged to initiate breastfeeding within the first hour. This time is also known as the 'golden hour,' a period of intense mutual gazing when infant and parent skin-to-skin contact stimulates the release of hormones facilitating breastfeeding and bonding.

The initial milk, also known as colostrum, is produced at this early stage. Colostrum, often referred to as 'liquid gold,' is a thick, yellowish substance teeming with antibodies and nutrients designed to give your newborn a healthy start. It's concentrated nutrition perfect for your newborn's tiny stomach.

4.2. Understanding the Latch

An effective latch is crucial for successful breastfeeding. It determines the flow of milk from breast to baby and plays a significant role in determining the comfort of the breastfeeding parent. If the latch is incorrect, it can lead to nipple soreness and low milk supply.

When it comes to securing a good latch, aim to bring the baby to the breast rather than the breast to the baby. The baby's mouth needs to cover not just the nipple but as much of the areola as possible. Don't be afraid to seek assistance from a lactation consultant or trained healthcare professional to ensure that you're on the right track.

4.3. The Production of Milk

In those early days, your body is hard at work figuring out precisely how much milk to produce. Success lies in the straightforward axiom—supply meets demand. The more frequently and efficiently your baby nurses, the more milk your body is signaled to produce.

The production of milk works in two stages:

1. Milk Ejection Reflex: This is signalled by the hormone oxytocin, causing muscle cells surrounding the alveoli where milk is stored to contract and release milk into the ducts leading to the nipple.

2. Milk Production: Prolactin, another hormone, regulates the actual production of milk inside the alveoli. With each feed, the level of prolactin in the blood increases, signalling the breasts to make more milk for the next feed.

When it comes to breastfeeding, frequent nursing is encouraged. It's completely normal for a newborn to want to nurse every two to three hours around the clock.

4.4. Navigating Growth Spurts

As the weeks pass, you might notice certain days where your baby seems hungrier, asking for more frequent feeds. These are known as 'growth spurts.' Common growth spurt times are around 2-3 weeks, 4-6 weeks, three months, and six months.

During these times, continue to feed on demand, as the frequent nursing will again signal your body's milk supply to increase. These spurts usually last a few days.

4.5. Introduction to Solids

The World Health Organization recommends exclusive breastfeeding until six months of age. After this, parents can start to introduce solid foods while continuing to breastfeed. This transition isn't always linear and requires patience.

Try introducing one food at a time, to observe the baby's response and identify any potential allergies. Grain cereals, fruits, and boiled, mashed vegetables are common first foods. Remember, the goal is to supplement breast milk, not replace it. The breast milk or formula should still constitute the major part of the baby's diet.

4.6. Weaning

The process of weaning, that is, transitioning from breast milk to other sources of nutrition, is highly individualized. The ages at which it happens differ from baby to baby. The AAP recommends breastfeeding for at least 12 months, and then as long after as both parent and baby wish.

There's no hard-set rule to how one should wean. Gradual weaning is often less stressful for both parent and baby. You might decide to drop one feeding session at a time. Over a period, your body will adjust to produce less milk, making the transition easier for both of you.

Breastfeeding is a transformative journey, one strewn with moments of doubt, joy, exhaustion, and profound love. From the first latch to the final weaning moment, understanding each stage can make the journey smoother, strengthening an already powerful bond with your child. Whatever the challenges may be, remember that support is available, be it a lactifying consultant, healthcare professional, or breastfeeding support group. Your breastfeeding journey is uniquely yours to navigate and cherish.

Chapter 5. Balancing Act: Juggling Breastfeeding and Daily Life

Breastfeeding is not only a beautifully nurturing natural process but also a skill that, like any other, demands time, patience, and practice to master. In the hustle and bustle of everyday life, it can sometimes feel challenging to manage the demands of breastfeeding along with other responsibilities. However, rest assured that, with the right strategies, breastfeeding can very well be a seamless part of daily life.

5.1. The Dance of Multitasking

Balancing family, work, and breastfeeding can indeed be akin to a dance. It is about rhythm and harmony, where patience and time management play pivotal roles. Some days might be smoother than others, but each day brings progress. Remember, it's about finding what works for you and your baby.

Building a routine is crucial, but this routine should be flexible. Babies cannot tell time, and their needs can change day by day or even hour by hour. Regular skin-to-skin contact often encourages more predictable feeding, and it has the bonus benefit of being a loving bonding activity. Also, consider babywearing. A good baby carrier can allow you to feed and respond promptly, while you go along with your tasks hands-free.

5.2. Returning to Work: Preparations and Strategies

Returning to work after maternity leave involves a major transition not just for you, but also for your baby. Ensuring that it has the least disruptive effect on your baby's feeding routine is of paramount importance.

Firstly, consider starting early, and anticipate this transition while you are still on maternity leave. Begin by expressing and storing milk. This practice will provide a back-up for your caregiver to feed the baby in your absence.

Also worth considering is familiarizing your baby with bottle-feeding. However, be cautious as to when you introduce the bottle. Introducing it too soon may result in nipple confusion, while delaying it too much may lead to the baby refusing the bottle altogether. Conventional advice proposes any time between two to six weeks after birth.

When returning to work, have a transparent conversation with your employer about your need to express milk. Most companies, in compliance with the law, should provide an appropriate space and breaks for this. Allowing your colleagues to understand your commitment to breastfeeding might mean sharing your intentions with them, which can also help cultivate a supportive environment.

5.3. Maintaining Milk Supply

A significant concern among breastfeeding parents who juggle multiple commitments is maintaining milk supply. Remember, breast milk is produced on demand; the more the baby feeds, the more milk is produced.

To maintain supply, advise your caregiver not to feed your baby an hour or so before you return home from work so that you can nurse immediately after. Regular night feeds can also help keep up the supply, as prolactin levels—the hormone responsible for milk regulation—are highest at night.

5.4. Navigating Through Public Spaces

Breastfeeding in public may feel challenging initially due to stigma and societal norms. However, remember that breastfeeding is a natural process and your right. Many countries have laws that specifically protect breastfeeding in public, so do get acquainted with them.

Prepare yourself for breastfeeding in public by practising at home. Dress for convenience and comfort and research on family-friendly facilities in public places, such as nursing rooms in shopping malls.

Cultivating a positive mindset goes a long way. It is a personal decision and might not always feel comfortable, but know that you are contributing to normalizing breastfeeding.

5.5. Self-care and Support

While it is easy to get caught in the tussle of responsibilities, remember not to neglect yourself. Eating well, staying hydrated, and resting adequately can directly impact your milk production and overall wellbeing.

Seek a circle of supporters who respect your decisions and encourage you. Connecting with other breastfeeding parents can offer network and emotional support. There are numerous community organizations and online platforms where advice, experiences, and support are shared.

Finally, finding a balance is a journey, not a destination. What works one day may not work the next, so be gentle with yourself. The process of breastfeeding not only shapes the lifelong bond of love and care between you and your baby but also mirrors your strength and resilience as a nurturer, provider, and guardian. Above all, remember that every drop of breast milk counts and so do you and your well-being.

Chapter 6. The Emotional Rollercoaster: Managing Stress & Mood Changes

Breastfeeding is far from simply a physical act; it's, in fact, an emotional journey brimming with joys, anxieties, and continual adjustments. In this chapter, we delve into the concept of the emotional rollercoaster that many breastfeeding parents ride, exploring the ins and outs of managing stress and mood changes along their journey.

6.1. Emotional Challenges in the Early Days

In the early days of breastfeeding, new parents may experience a tumultuous mixture of emotions. A potent cocktail of hormones, sleep deprivation, and the sudden responsibility of caring for a new life can result in a bumpy ride. The Joy that a new life brings is often intermingled with feelings of insecurity, exhaustion, frustration, and anxiety. It is important to know that these feelings are perfectly normal and to remember that there is a vast support network available, ready to provide emotional and practical help.

The very act of breastfeeding can, in itself cause mood swings. This is due to the release of hormones such as oxytocin, also known as the 'love hormone', and prolactin during nursing. While these hormones help stimulate the flow of milk and enforce the maternal bond, they can also lead to feelings of deep calm one moment to tearfulness the next.

Biological factors are not solely to blame though. Cultural and societal pressures also contribute to the emotional challenges faced by parents in the early days of breastfeeding. The postpartum period is often rife with intense pressure to become the 'perfect parent' instantly, a wholly unrealistic expectation that can foster unhealthy guilt and self-doubt.

6.2. Understanding the Stress Response

Breastfeeding or chestfeeding parents may also experience moments of intense stress. Stress can manifest in various ways, from physical symptoms such as headaches or increased heart rate to more subtle indications like irritability or difficulty concentrating.

What causes stress for one person may not for another. Some breastfeeding parents might feel anxious about ensuring their baby is obtaining enough nutrition, while others might struggle with society's conflicting views on appropriate breastfeeding practice. Such stresses can strain or interrupt the relationship you are trying to forge with your baby.

However, understanding the stress response can help you manage it. When faced with a stressor, the body undergoes several changes: adrenaline is released, heart rate increases, and muscles tense up. These changes prepare the body for what is commonly known as 'fight or flight' mode. Recognizing that this response is a natural reaction designed to protect us can go a long way in helping manage the stress of breastfeeding.

6.3. Coping Strategies for Managing Stress and Mood Changes

Now that we understand the stress response and have acknowledged various sources of anxiety, let's discuss strategies to manage stress and mood changes effectively.

Exercise is an excellent tool for managing stress as it promotes the release of endorphins, the body's natural painkillers and mood elevators. Even simple routines like going for a walk, practicing gentle yoga, or performing basic maternity exercises can significantly help.

Other effective strategies include deep breathing exercises, mindfulness therapy, meditation, and visualization techniques. Each of these methods is designed to soothe the body and mind, helping you stay present during the breastfeeding process.

When dealing with mood swings and stress, it's essential to stay connected to your support network. It could comprise family, friends, lactation consultants, or local support groups. Be open and honest about your feelings and talk to someone you trust. Remember, there is no shame in seeking support, and often, a listening ear can provide immense comfort.

Proper nutrition and hydration during the postpartum period can also be a huge factor in managing mood changes. Eat balanced meals, incorporating foods rich in omega-3, proteins, vitamins, and minerals in your diet. Hydration aids the production of breast milk and can also improve your mood and energy levels.

6.4. Are Mood Changes a Sign of Something More?

Lastly, while it's completely normal to experience mood swings while breastfeeding, it's also crucial to be aware of when these changes might signal something more serious. If feelings of sadness, anxiety, or hopelessness last more than two weeks or feel overwhelming, this could be a sign of postpartum depression. This is a serious condition affecting one in seven parents after birth and requires immediate medical attention.

It's of utmost importance that, as a breastfeeding parent, you are aware of these risks and remember that seeking help is not a sign of weakness but a testament to your strength and dedication to your wellbeing and, ultimately, your baby's happiness.

As we concluded this chapter, the truth stands that breastfeeding, like any profound human experience, involves its fair share of stress and mood changes. But with understanding, strategies in place, and an open line to a community of support, you can navigate this emotional rollercoaster successfully and relish the intimacy, bonding, and deep love that this journey offers.

Chapter 7. Addressing Common Challenges: From Latching Issues to Low Supply

Breastfeeding can be an enriching adventure for both parent and child, but it often comes with its own set of challenges. Some parents may struggle with latching difficulties, some may grapple with low milk supply. No worry is too small or too large during this intimate process. That's why this part is centered around addressing these common challenges.

7.1. Latching Issues

Latching is the process whereby the baby attaches or 'latches' onto the breast to nurse. A proper latch is elemental to successful breastfeeding, ensuring the baby is able to draw enough milk and that the breastfeeding parent is not caused undue discomfort.

Many parents may encounter difficulties with latching at first. Although it is a natural process, it doesn't always come naturally. However, with time, patience, and a bit of professional guidance, these obstacles can usually be overcome.

The most common indicator of latching difficulties is pain while nursing. If it continues post-feed or after the first week of breastfeeding, it's time to get help. Flat or inverted nipples, nipple soreness, and blanched, cracked, or bleeding nipples can be other signs of improper latching.

There are a variety of methods which can be utilized to overcome latching issues:

1. Seek professional help: A lactation consultant can provide invaluable support and guidance, helping to establish a comfortable and efficient latch.

2. Experiment with holds: Different positions might work best for different dyads. Some popular breastfeeding positions include cradle hold, football hold, and laid-back breastfeeding or biological nurturing.

3. Provide skin-to-skin contact: Skin-to-skin can encourage instinctual behaviors and assist with the establishment of an efficient latch.

4. Ensure baby opens mouth wide: A wide mouth indicates the baby is ready to latch. It may be beneficial to wait for this sign before bringing the baby onto the breast.

5. Repeat at every feed: Persistence is key. If a latch is painful, unlatch (by inserting a clean finger into the corner of baby's mouth to break the suction) and try again.

7.2. Low Milk Supply

Another challenge which may arise during breastfeeding is the concern over low milk supply. It's important to remember that the majority of breastfeeding parents can produce enough milk for their babies. In fact, the principle of supply and demand dictates milk formation - the more your baby nurses, the more milk you will produce. However, there can be complicated factors at play, and sometimes, perceived low supply can lead to stress and worry.

The signs of low milk supply may include poor or slow weight gain, infrequent or dark-colored urine and stools in the baby, and a decrease in breast fullness or leaking. If you are unsure whether or not your supply is adequate, consulting a pediatrician or lactation consultant can provide much-needed reassurance or advice.

Here are some strategies to manage concerns of low milk supply:

1. Nurse on demand: Allow your baby to nurse whenever they show signs of hunger. Quickened movements, awake and calm state, head turning, and hands to mouth are hunger cues to look for.

2. Maintain skin-to-skin: Like with latching, skin-to-skin contact helps promote nursing behavior and can encourage more frequent feeds, thereby possibly increasing milk supply.

3. Incorporate healthy habits: Staying hydrated, eating balanced meals, and getting as much rest as possible can support your body in maintaining or increasing milk production.

4. Utilize breast compressions: This strategy involves applying gentle pressure on the breast while nursing, encouraging more efficient transfer of milk to the baby.

5. Use lactation aids: Many breastfeeding parents find herbal galactagogues like fenugreek, moringa, or blessed thistle helpful for boosting milk supply, though these should be used under professional guidance.

Remember, each breastfeeding journey is unique, and it's okay to seek help and support when necessary. Through understanding common challenges like latching issues and low milk supply, we hope to empower you with the knowledge needed to navigate these hurdles with confidence and grace. After all, a well-supported breastfeeding parent can be a crucial element to their child's thriving start in life.

Chapter 8. Breastfeeding Benefits: Going Beyond Nutrition

It is through our earliest contacts with our world that we begin gathering the foundational experiences that shape us into who we are. Among these, breastfeeding stands out as a unique interaction. It is primarily perceived as a simple act of nourishment yet in truth, it goes way beyond just feeding. It is a symbiotic conversation between the parent and the infant, an immersion into intense bonding, nurturing love, and developing immense psychological and physiological benefits for both.

8.1. Understanding Breastfeeding

Breastfeeding begins with the first suckle of breastmilk, a superfood tailored by nature. It is a concoction of numerous nutrients, including proteins, fats, sugars, vitamins and more, combined with the mother's immune factors and enzymes. Unique to each dyad, breastmilk shifts and modifies its contents in response to the baby's needs. But despite its nutritional credentials, breastfeeding is not merely about providing sustenance. The act itself weaves in benefits that reach into the psychological, emotional, and physiological realms.

8.2. Psychological and Emotional Benefits for the Child

Research has long proclaimed the value of skin-to-skin contact between parent and child in the early days. It has shown to contribute significantly to the psychological and emotional development of the child. Breastfeeding amplifies such encounters by multiplying the chances for contact, inextricably linking the baby's feeding time with a strong sense of comfort, safety, and closeness.

Breastfeeding has also been seen to facilitate secure attachment patterns in the child. Quite simply, a securely attached child trusts that their needs will be met promptly and lovingly. This trust provides a solid base from which they can explore the world, fostering high self-esteem, and offering better resilience in the face of adversity.

In addition, breastfeeding spawns numerous emotional benefits for the child. Along with secure attachment, the act of breastfeeding helps the child better manage their emotions, instilling a sense of calm and reducing instances of aggressive or distress-like behaviour.

8.3. Psychological and Emotional Benefits for the Parent

The advantages of breastfeeding extend to the parents as well. Nurturing a child by breastfeeding instils a sense of empowerment and confidence. The knowledge that they are not just feeding but significantly contributing to the overall well-being of their child can boost a parent's self-confidence and reduce feelings of anxiety, doubt, or fear often experienced during early parenthood.

Breastfeeding also engenders a sense of deep-seated connection with the baby, an unspoken communication that fortifies emotional bonds. Each breastfeeding session is an opportunity for the parents to slow down, relax, and revel in the shared quiet with the infant, facilitating mindfulness and helping reduce postnatal depression.

8.4. Physical Benefits for the Child

Scientific and health organizations across the globe unanimously support breastfeeding, primarily due to its innumerate physical health benefits for the child. It is associated with lower incidences of childhood illnesses such as ear infections, respiratory ailments, gastrointestinal disturbances, and more.

Breastfeeding has also shown beneficial in immunological programming, providing the child with an immunological armor derived from the parent's immune system. Furthermore, breastfeeding has protective effects against the development of later life non-communicable diseases like obesity, type 2 diabetes, and cardiovascular diseases.

8.5. Physical Benefits for the Parent

Physical health benefits are not restricted to the child alone; significant gains have been observed for the parents as well. Exclusive breastfeeding can help in quicker postpartum healing, with lesser risks of postpartum hemorrhaging. It also assists in natural weight-loss post childbirth due to the additional calorie expenditure involved in milk synthesis.

Breastfeeding's health benefits extend long after the act has ceased. It lowers the risk of breast and ovarian cancers, reduces the chances of developing rheumatoid arthritis, cardiovascular ailments, and type 2 diabetes, providing protective effects that can endure over the years.

8.6. Understanding the Extended Benefits

While the tangible benefits of breastfeeding are widely recognized, there are myriad extended and relational perks that can be linked to the practice. For instance, breastfeeding encourages the development of the child's oral cavity, playing a crucial role in facilitating proper speech development and alignment of teeth.

Simultaneously, in societies often embroiled in environmental discussions, breastfeeding emerges as an environmentally friendly practice. It obviates the need for bottles, teats, formula cans, and other paraphernalia associated with formula feeding, reducing waste and conserving resources.

In conclusion, breastfeeding triumphs as a powerful link between the mother and the child, one which is not just nutritive but imbued with intense physical, emotional and psychological bonding. Its role in building a healthy society is underscored by the fact that its benefits transcend generations, leaving imprints that linger through the lifetime of an individual, and even beyond. It is an unparalleled act where natural biology and profound love intertwines, creating a nurturing world for Parent and Child, while ensuring an invaluable legacy for the generations to come.

Chapter 9. Support Systems: Building Your Breastfeeding Network

Building a support system for your breastfeeding journey is a crucial step that can greatly enhance your overall experience. Receiving valuable guidance, encouragement, and help from a variety of resources can boost not only your knowledge but also your confidence. Hence, this chapter aims at providing you with a detailed guide on constructing your personal network.

9.1. Trusted Healthcare Professionals

On top of your breastfeeding network are healthcare professionals who carry essential knowledge about the process. Your obstetrician, pediatrician, and especially a lactation consultant should be the first points of contact.

Lactation consultants are specialists trained in breastfeeding and are equipped to help manage common issues such as latching difficulties, painful nursing, and low milk production. They are a rich source of accurate, practical information and emotional support. Make sure to select a lactation consultant who is board-certified to ensure the best advice.

Moreover, regular pediatric care is essential to monitor your child's growth and development, and pediatricians can often provide breastfeeding support, especially regarding your child's health, growth, and the pharmacology of breastfeeding.

9.2. Experienced Family and Friends

Having family and friends who have already been through the process can provide realistic insights, practical tips, troubleshooting, and most importantly, emotional bolstering. While professional advice is important, personal experiences shared by loved ones add a priceless value to your journey.

It's beneficial to reach out to these individuals early, ideally during pregnancy, to solicit their insights. Don't hesitate to ask even the simplest of questions as, often, it's these little details that pave the way for a smoother experience.

9.3. Breastfeeding Support Groups and Online Forums

These groups can be a prolific source of support and encouragement, allowing you to openly share your concerns and receive valuable advice from parents who are at various stages of their own breastfeeding journeys.

Numerous local and national organizations offer gatherings, including La Leche League International. These groups also often provide hotlines for instant support. Online platforms, where you can post queries anytime, also prove helpful. However, it's important to cross-verify any information gathered from online sources with your healthcare provider.

9.4. Self-Education: Books and Online Resources

This is where your self-study comes in. Numerous books written by breastfeeding experts can offer in-depth knowledge, practical tips, and potential solutions to hurdles. 'The Womanly Art of Breastfeeding' by Diane Wiessinger, 'Breastfeeding Made Simple' by Nancy Mohrbacher and Kathleen Kendall-Tackett, and 'The Breastfeeding Book' by Martha Sears are few of many such resources.

Online educational resources, podcasts, webinars, videos, and blogs can provide quick, digestible bits of valuable knowledge. Some reliable online platforms include KellyMom, the Australian Breastfeeding Association's website, and the American Academy of Pediatrics' breastfeeding page.

9.5. Personal Mindset and Self-Care

Your approach towards breastfeeding, including your emotional wellbeing, carries significant importance. The journey can be exhausting, overwhelming, and seemingly endless during the early days. Here, understanding the process, being patient with yourself and your baby, and taking care of your mental health by practicing mindfulness, or engaging in relaxing activities can do wonders. Engaging a professional for mental health support can also be considered.

Breastfeeding is a symbol and cultural practice of deep love, care, and bonding. The journey is unique, and each person's experience differs. Having a strong, diverse support network is highly beneficial for making it a successful, satisfying, and rewarding experience. Remember, support is not one-size-fits-all; pick and choose what best suits you and your baby. This is your journey – embrace it in your own unique way!

Chapter 10. Nurturing Yourself While Nurturing Your Baby: Self-care During Breastfeeding

Breastfeeding is an intimate journey, a profound act of nurturing, and bonding that sets the stage for a lifetime of maternal-infant connectivity. At the same time, it is a demanding experience, physically and emotionally. Incorporating self-care amidst this journey is crucial to ensuring both your wellbeing and your baby's. While you focus on feeding and caring for your newborn, you should not lose sight of your wellbeing.

10.1. Incorporating Rest and Sleep

Breastfeeding is inherently energy-consuming. It may sometimes feel as though you're running on empty, especially in the first few weeks following delivery when your baby feeds around the clock. Here, prioritizing rest is important. Try to rest while your baby is sleeping, even if it's a brief nap in the day.

It might be tempting to use this time to catch up on chores, but remember that your body is in recovery mode and needs all the rest it can get. Certainly, keeping a tidy home is important, but it's okay to let a few things slide during these early weeks. Your focus should be recuperating and gaining strength, so you are better placed to care for your baby.

10.2. Eating Right

During the process of breastfeeding, your body is working to produce milk while recovering from childbirth. Maintaining a healthy diet can thus help replenish nutrients, boost milk production, and aid recovery. Include plenty of fruits, vegetables, whole grains, and protein-rich foods in your meals.

Ensuring you eat regularly is as important as the quality of food you consume. Plan your meals and snacks ahead of time to mitigate the risk of skipping meals. Store healthy, grab-and-go snacks near your breastfeeding station for times when you're unable to prepare something to eat, making sure to avoid overly processed, high-sugar snacks.

10.3. Hydration During Breastfeeding

Breast milk is approximately 90% water. As a breastfeeding parent, you'll likely notice an increased thirst. During each feeding, it might be helpful to have a glass of water to resplenish your hydration level. Avoid excessive intake of caffeinated beverages and alcohol as they can have dehydrating effects.

10.4. Exercise and Movement

Breastfeeding or not, regular physical exercise is beneficial for overall health. In the postpartum period, light exercises like walking or gentle yoga can aid recovery, promote mood stability, and improve energy levels. However, it's crucial to listen to your body and consult with your healthcare provider before starting any physical activity regimen.

10.5. Emotional Wellbeing

Breastfeeding is a journey that comes with a myriad of emotions - overwhelming love, fatigue, doubt, joy, anxiety, and more. It's natural for these feelings to ebb and flow. Emotional health isn't simply about feeling good all the time—it's about recognizing your feelings, understanding that it's okay to have a variety of emotions, and not hesitating to seek help when needed.

Joining a breastfeeding support group can be beneficial in managing the emotional journey. Connecting with other breastfeeding parents might provide reassurance, generate useful tips, and remind you that you're not alone. Also, consider discussing your feelings with your healthcare provider if feelings of depression or anxiety persist.

10.6. Time for Yourself

In the whirlwind that is new parenthood, it's easy to lose oneself. Carving out time for self-care, no matter how little, can go a long way in keeping your spirits up. It could be as simple as reading a few pages of a book, enjoying a cup of tea, meditating, or having a relaxing bath. Remember, you can ask for help from your partner, family, or friends to find that valuable 'me time'.

Breastfeeding is a commitment. In fulfilling this commitment, your health and wellbeing should not be sacrificed. By integrating self-care into your life, you build resilience, rejuvenate your energy, and cultivate a holistic sense of wellbeing pivotal in sustaining the breastfeeding journey. It equips you to love, care for, and nurture your baby to the best of your ability, for cycles of love and nurturing are fueled when the nurturer is nourished. Your parenting journey, after all, should be balanced with self-nurture, empowering you to be both a loving parent and a happy individual.

Chapter 11. The Art of Weaning: Transitioning with Love and Patience

Breastfeeding, for many, is a period of deep connection and intimacy between a parent and child. While it is a magical journey that both the parent and the baby embark upon, the path can be filled with trials, surprises, and rewards. One such significant and challenging milestone on this journey is the process of weaning.

Weaning, in the simplest of terms, is the gradual introduction of foods other than breast milk into a baby's diet. It signifies a major transition for both the breastfeeding parent and child. A well-paced and mindful approach can make this significant transition smoother, nurturing and loving, mirroring the breastfeeding experience.

11.1. Understanding Weaning

Weaning is not merely a transition from breast milk to solid foods, but a phase where a child learns to give up something familiar and comforting. It's more than just a nutrition-based transition; it's a relationship and emotional shift. Understanding its significance forms the first step towards weaning with love and patience.

Weaning can be initiated naturally by the child – known as child-led weaning, or by the parent - termed as parent-led weaning. Child-led weaning often occurs when the child is ready, somewhere between the ages of 1-2 years. In parent-led weaning, due to various reasons such as returning to work or other lifestyle factors, a parent might decide to initiate the process earlier.

11.2. Signs Your Child Is Ready for Weaning

Every child is unique; the readiness to wean could appear as early as 4 months or as late as 2 years. Recognizing the signs can ease the transition. Some indications include demonstrated curiosity in solid food, ability to sit upright unassisted, decreased nursing frequency, and teething.

A sudden unexplained decrease in nursing often referred to as a 'nursing strike,' however, is not necessarily an indication of readiness for weaning. It might be attributed to teething, ear infection, or even a change in the nursing environment.

11.3. Starting the Weaning Process

Patience and a gradual approach are key when initiating weaning. It can be helpful to start by substituting one feed at a time, beginning with the least preferred one by the baby.

Introducing a varied range of flavors and textures during the initial stages of weaning could help prevent a fussy palate later. Ensure the foods are age-appropriate, and remember, the initial goal is to help a child familiarize themselves with solid food rather than count on it for nutrition. Gradually start increasing the quantity and variety as the baby gets comfortable.

Maintain the intimacy of breastfeeding during weaning. Co-nurse, if possible, ensuring that the time spent during these meals is calm, comfortable, and pleasurable for both of you.

11.4. Emotional Component of Weaning

The emotional aspects of weaning can be as intense for the breastfeeding parent as for the child. Feelings of relief, sadness, guilt, and liberation can all surface during this transition. Constant reassurance of love may be required for the child as they navigate this unfamiliar terrain.

Remember, it's more of the nourishing relationship than the milk itself that a child might miss. Substitute nursing time with reading, cuddling, or simply spending quality time to signal that your bond is not exclusively tied to breastfeeding.

11.5. Dealing with Weaning Resistance

Resistance towards weaning can occur due to various reasons - the child might be feeling unwell, or there could be big changes like a move or a new sibling. Be patient and flexible during such times. If resistance continues, it might be worthwhile to pause and revisit weaning later.

11.6. Expert Support and Peer Sharing

Don't hesitate to reach out for help. Pediatricians, lactation consultants, and support groups could provide invaluable guidance during this transition.

Weaning, like breastfeeding, can be a beautiful shared experience between a parent and child with the right approach. As you embark on this journey, remember to trust your instincts, validate your child's feelings, and be guided by love and patience. The art of weaning, therefore, is not just about introducing solid food, but nurturing a growing independence while maintaining the warmth of your bond. Seek support, share experiences, and most importantly, celebrate this significant milestone together.

www.ingramcontent.com/pod-product-compliance
Lightning Source LLC
Chambersburg PA
CBHW060900260726
48661CB00008B/3371